Compassionate Kombucha

How to Brew Your Own for Healing and Manifestation

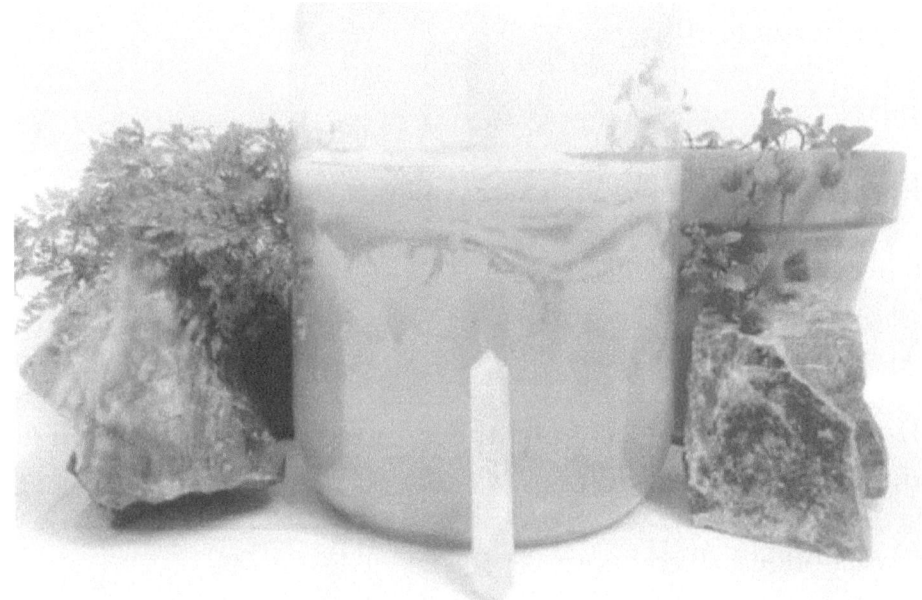

By Allison Gee

First Printing: 2015

ISBN   978-1-329-10006-0

Printed in the United States of America.

Cover Design by Allison Gee

You are reading Edition 1

If you would like to contact the author, please visit Allison at the following web address:

www.goddessallison.com

Table of Contents

By Allison Gee

Introduction

Brewing Kombucha can be easy and fun. Consuming Kombucha can have many benefits. If you would like to drink Kombucha regularly, it can be a great skill to learn how to brew your own.

In this helpful guidebook we will get into the brewing basics for this delicious tonic. Brewing the drink itself is simple and requires few ingredients. It is important to become proficient in the basics of brewing before you add extra ingredients and experiment with utilizing this drink for healing and manifestation.

After the brewing basics we will talk about the health benefits of Kombucha, and you will learn how to use it as a healing tool. Kombucha is a fermented drink and can assist you in healing a wide variety of ailments. The drink is considered a probiotic and is helpful for maintaining healthy intestinal flora. When your body is healthy, your immune system strengthens and your cells regenerate to overcome many adverse conditions.

After the health benefits we will talk about using this magical elixir as a companion in manifestation. Using a drink to attain more money, love, and anything you desire may be a revolutionary concept for some, but legends of love potions will no longer be a fictional fantasy in your life after reading this book. For many, the information presented here is common knowledge, but this may be the first time you have been gifted this knowledge specifically about Kombucha.

May the pages of this gift open your life to the secrets of sages and sorcerers.

Medical Disclaimer: The information in this book has not been approved by the FDA and is not designed to diagnose, treat, cure, or prevent disease in accordance with the standards of the United States Food and Drug Administration. This information is not being provided to you by a licensed medical or health care professional. It is the reader's sole responsibility for any risk or benefit incurred after following the guidance presented in this publication, and by reading this book you agree to accept that responsibility and liability.

Author's Disclaimer: The information about Kombucha, presented in this book, may never be approved by the FDA as an acceptable substance for healing. Nature, herbs, tea, healthy yeast and bacteria, water, sugar, and your own infusion of imagination are not considered patentable, marketable healing substances by FDA standards. Although there is no strong scientific evidence from the United States that supports the use of Kombucha in healing ailments, there is also no strong evidence from the FDA that there are any adverse side effects in utilizing Kombucha as a food. It is safe to consume, provided that your brew remains healthy.

According to many standards in the current structures of the medical industry, science, and spirituality of the United States of America, it may be absurd for any one of them to prescribe the intake of Kombucha for healing and manifestation. This advice is being provided to you by a manifestation mentor who has over a decade of experience and education in the holistic field. You are welcome to take it or leave it.

Compassionate Kombucha

Brewing Basics

Brewing Kombucha requires a few main ingredients so it is important to acquire these ingredients before you get started. Even if you are an experienced Kombucha brewer, you will benefit from reading this chapter. We will go into detail for each ingredient, but here is a list of the main ingredients:

Scoby + Starter Tea

Tea

Sugar

Water

You will also need:

A Container

A Cloth Cover

A Rubber Band

It's that simple! So, you want to brew some Kombucha right now!?

First you will need a container to house your new pet. Growing Kombucha comes with responsibility and empowerment so it is important to start out with a compassionate heart, as if you were welcoming home a new pet (it may be the only kind of pet you can have if you live in a dwelling where "pets" are not allowed). When acquiring ingredients for brewing Kombucha, it is important to have the most pure and healthy (for instance, buy organic tea instead of generic tea).

A Container

It is recommended that you use a glass or ceramic container for your Kombucha. It is a fermented food so metal and plastic containers are not advisable. A wide mouthed glass jar works very well. You may need to attain two different containers if you want to build up to brewing a large amount of Kombucha. For instance, start with a pint or quart jar, and also acquire a gallon jar for your next brew.

Never use soap to clean your Kombucha container. Instead use hot water, vinegar, and a splash of lemon juice. Soap is not good for the health of your brew.

Scoby + Starter Tea

Before you start your brew, you will need to attain a Scoby. This is a live culture of helpful yeast and bacteria that is specifically used for brewing Kombucha. A Scoby is not actually considered to be a mushroom or an algae, but several of its nicknames from many cultures have described it as such. The Scoby is also called "the mother" because it produces more of itself. Utilizing an organism that freely

6

produces more of itself is a powerful analogy for manifestation. If you know someone who brews Kombucha you can attain a Scoby from them. If you do not have personal access to a Kombucha brewer, you may order a Scoby from the internet or grow one yourself using the right commercial Kombucha.

Your Scoby should come in some starter tea. This is brewed Kombucha from a previous batch. The amount of Kombucha you create with your first batch should correspond with the amount of starter tea you acquire. See the Ratios in the Brewing Instructions section of this chapter for more information. If you do not receive starter tea with your Scoby, you can either purchase commercial Kombucha or you can use white distilled vinegar or apple cider vinegar.

It is ideal to attain a Scoby and starter tea that came from a healthy brew of Kombucha. If you are not able to deduce the health of the brew from which you are receiving your ingredients (your new pet), it is best to order one from a reputable source and start there. You will strengthen the health of your Scoby and brew using the information in this book. Make sure that the Scoby you are ordering is fresh. Do not order a dehydrated Scoby.

If you purchase commercial Kombucha to grow a starter Scoby or use it for starter tea, make sure it has not been pasteurized, flavored, or reformulated. It should be pure 100% plain Kombucha. To cause it to grow a Scoby, just leave it out for a couple weeks. Do not refrigerate it, even if it says to do so on the bottle, and make sure there is a large surface area on top of the liquid. Transfer the liquid to another container if you need to because the Scoby will form on the surface of the liquid.

<u>Tea</u>

It is advisable to use Green Tea or Black Tea to brew your Kombucha. You can use other herbal teas but you may risk jeopardizing the health of your brew until you gain more experience as a brewer. I will give more detailed information on tea types in the Healing and Manifestation chapters, but if you are a beginner at brewing, just start with Green Tea or Black Tea. You will need to grow a large healthy Scoby to start experimenting with other teas. Your final brew will taste different than the original tea flavor, so don't expect that your Kombucha will taste like the tea does after it is steeped.

Green Tea brews into a Kombucha with a light, refreshing taste.

Black Tea brews into a Kombucha with an earthy taste.

You can decide which kind of tea you'd like to use. My favorite is Jasmine Green Tea and fruity Green

Teas like blueberry. It's important to make sure your tea does not have any artificial flavors or additives. If you want fruit flavored tea, it's best to buy the organic dried form of the fruit and combine it with the pure loose leaf form of Green or Black Tea.

In order to deduce a favorable tea for yourself you can try the following exercise:

Tea Buying Exercise~ In order to be an effective manifestor, it is important to utilize an acute intuition. If you are a beginner at using your intuition, this exercise will help you hone your own internal compass. It may sound simple or silly, but just go with it. Go to the store; preferably one with a large tea selection. While you are in the tea section, literally ask yourself either out loud or inside your head,

"Which tea shall I buy in order for me to brew the highest and best Kombucha for my body and my life?"

Ask yourself over and over a few times if necessary, and just stand there in the aisle to see what jumps out at your attention. Resist the urge to think or analyze your tea choice. This is meant to be a fun experiment for you to see what kind of tea you come up with. If it is not based in Green or Black Tea, buy it anyway and purchase a simple straight Green or Black Tea in addition to the one your intuition and imagination picked out. You will use this tea after you have brewed a few successful batches with the Green or

Black. If you are an experienced Kombucha brewer, this is a fun exercise to try and start brewing your tea right away, using part of your mother Scoby for a new batch.

Sugar

It is best to use either white cane sugar or organic cane juice crystals to brew your Kombucha, especially if you are a beginner at brewing.

Brown sugar is not advisable because it contains molasses and can be hard on the Scoby to process the extra nutrients.

You can use honey or agave, but this is not advisable for beginning brewers. The batch results with honey and agave can be inconsistent or possibly jeopardize the health of your brew so this method of sweetener is only advised for experienced brewers. If you are an experienced brewer, it is best to have a healthy Scoby as a back up before you start experimenting with these sweeteners.

You can use maple syrup, but it must be organic and have no extra ingredients. You can use it at a ratio of 1/2-2/3 of the amount of cane sugar you would use.

Do not use stevia and do not use synthetic or highly processed sweeteners like high fructose corn syrup and xylitol. They do not contain the nutrients your Scoby needs to thrive.

The purpose of adding sugar to your batch is so that your Scoby can grow, thrive, and turn the sugars into a fermented vinegary, CO_2, and ethanol (alcohol) mixture. This is a fermented drink and there are only very small trace amounts of sugar and naturally occurring alcohol in your final brew so this is nothing to be concerned about if you are cautions of your sugar or alcohol intake. This is not considered an alcoholic drink and you will not feel effects from drinking Kombucha as you would other sugary or alcoholic drinks. The sugar is for your Scoby to eat, not for you, so it is important to follow the ratios of sugar when making your batch. If you use less sugar than the 1 cup to 1 gallon ratio, you are starving your Scoby or making it harder for it to thrive.

Water

It is important to use the most pure, clean water you can to brew your Kombucha. Use filtered water, spring water, or distilled water. If you only have access to potable tap water, it's best to let the water sit for about 12-24 hours before you heat it up to brew your tea. Because you will be boiling the water for tea anyway, tap water is an acceptable ingredient if you have nothing else.

Brewing Instructions

Ratios. Use these ratios when creating your brew:

1 Quart : 2 tea bags or 1.5 tsp loose leaf : 1/4 cup sugar : 2-3 cups water : 1/2 cup starter tea.

1/2 Gallon : 4 tea bags or 1 tbs loose leaf : 1/2 cup sugar : 6-7 cups water : 1 cup starter tea.

1 Gallon : 8 tea bags or 2 tbs loose leaf : 1 cup sugar : 13-14 cups water : 2 cups starter tea.

Decide where your brewing Kombucha will live.

Many Kombucha brewing sources may say to store your brew in a dark cupboard, but personally, I do not like the idea of shutting my Kombucha into a cupboard. You probably wouldn't shut your pet into a cupboard. Pets need attention, and people are likely to forget about things shut into cupboards or hidden away in dark places.

Many sources also say you need to store Kombucha in a warm dark place, but this may not necessarily be true. Sometimes warm dark places don't have enough air circulation for a healthy brew and you risk growing mold. You don't need to put it into a cupboard, but avoid bright light or direct sunlight and avoid extreme heat or cold. Kombucha thrives at around 70-80 degrees F (21-26 degrees C), so a warm dimly lit place will do just fine. Make sure it is out somewhere you will see it and pay attention to it often. This is important for compassionate Kombucha.

Heat your water. If you are using Black Tea, bring the water to a boil. If you are using Green Tea bring the water to a rolling simmer. The water does not need to be as hot for Green Tea. If you are using another type of tea, it is helpful to know the optimal water temperature for the type you are using. If you want to get technical, you can use a cooking thermometer, but it isn't necessary.

Convenient ways of heating water for the avid brewer are: a hot water spigot on the faucet specifically for dispensing water hotter than the regular tap, an electric kettle, and some refrigerators or other machines will directly dispense hot water that can be used to make tea.

Add your tea. Let your tea steep for 5-10 minutes. Steep for less time for Green Tea and more time for Black Tea. Then you will need to remove the tea. Use a strainer if you choose to put the loose leaf tea directly into the hot water.

Add the sugar. Adding the sugar while the tea is still hot makes it easier to dissolve, but adding the Scoby while the tea is still hot is not a good idea. It may hurt or damage your healthy Scoby. If you want to put the Scoby into the tea right away, it is a good idea to stir in some ice cubes to bring the water temperature down. It is also a good idea to just leave the tea to cool to room temperature and go do something else before adding the Scoby.

Add the Scoby + Starter Tea. Make sure you pour the tea into your brewing container before adding the Scoby and starter tea. If your Scoby does not float right away, this is all right. As the Kombucha brews, the Scoby will float to the top or a new Scoby will form on the surface and conform to your new container.

At this stage in the re-brewing process (when your Scoby is already in your brewing container), I find it helpful to tilt the container and pour the newly brewed sweet tea in along the edge of the Scoby. This way, the Scoby stays afloat and you save some energy from taking it out and putting it back in again. If you would like to take the Scoby out, you can set it on a clean plate while you pour and stir in your freshly steeped tea. Make sure you are practicing impeccable hygiene through the process.

Cover your brew. There should be at least 2-3 inches of space between your cover and the surface of your brew to allow for air circulation. Use the cloth to cover the opening on your container, and use the rubber band to secure it. It is nice for the Scoby if the cloth is large enough to hang over the sides and shield the Scoby from the light when you are using a clear glass jar. Use an impermeable cloth because if you use a mesh cloth, like cheese cloth, it may be possible for pests, like fruit flies, to infest your brew. Some people wish to cover their brew with a lid to increase carbonation, but a thriving Scoby needs good air circulation, so it is not a good idea to lid your brew long term.

Brew! Let your brew work its magic for about 7 to 14 days. If you are not familiar with your own preferences for taste and sweetness, do a taste test at 7, 10, and 14 days to see which brewing time you like the best. Ideally a compassionate Kombucha brewer would pay attention to their Scoby every day~ Talk to it and tell it how much you love and appreciate it. Thank it. Send it blessings, prayers, and good vibes.

Enjoy! When your brew is done, savor and enjoy this delicious tonic. Share it with others, and spread the compassionate Kombucha love. I have found it makes a great addition to potlucks. It's also a great conversation piece for curious guests. Don't forget to leave enough tea to start your next batch. You can use your Scoby, ideally indefinitely, as it will grow new layers each time you brew. After 4 to 5 brews, you can peel old layers away and either compost them, give them to a friend, or experiment with a new manifesting potion.

Troubleshooting

Brown Film. A brown film may develop on your Scoby or on the bottom of the container. This is normal and can be brushed off or strained out. It is safe to eat.

Mold. Do not use moldy layers of Scoby. This only happens in warm dark places that do not get enough air circulation. Ideally a compassionate Kombucha brewer would be paying attention to their brew often so mold would not grow.

If you notice mold, you may need to move your brew to a different location- one that is cooler and has better air circulation. Peel away and discard moldy layers, rinse your Scoby well, and start a new brew. If you are squeamish, you can start over all together.

Pests. Fruit flies love Kombucha and will fly into your brew and lay eggs if they get the chance. This is why it is so important to keep it covered with an impermeable cloth.

If you have too many fruit flies in your house you can make a trap for them with some Kombucha. Put Kombucha in the bottom of a container with a narrow opening. Cover the opening with a funnel or a funnel-shaped piece of paper. They will fly in and be trapped.

Going on Vacation. Kombucha can live for 2-3 months unattended. Your brew will be vinegar by then but you can use it for anything you would normally use vinegar for, like cooking or cleaning. If you need to be away for more than a few weeks, you can also find a trusted friend or family member to take care of it while you are gone. If you need to be away from your Kombucha brew for more than 2 months, you can make it slow down by putting it into the refrigerator. Refrigeration of a brewing batch can be used as a last resort but is not recommended. It will take a few brewing cycles for a refrigerated Scoby to return to its regular thriving, brewing state.

Refrigeration. It is not necessary to refrigerate brewing Kombucha and it is not recommended that you refrigerate the Scoby. The only reason you would want to refrigerate Kombucha liquid is to drastically slow down the brewing process and prevent it from growing a Scoby before you wish to drink it. The reason commercial Kombucha needs to be refrigerated is because it often contains other ingredients, like fruit juice. The brewer also wants to keep it from brewing through packaging, transportation, and shelf life as well as comply with health code policies surrounding food. Commercial Kombucha is considered a "perishable item," but you may never need to refrigerate your own homegrown Kombucha.

Compassionate Kombucha

By Allison Gee

Kombucha for Health and Healing

Kombucha has been used for thousands of years in many parts of the world as a drink that promotes longevity, good health, and healing. There is currently no strong "scientific" or "medical" evidence in the United States of America that Kombucha does miraculous things, like helps to cure cancer and viruses. The United States of America is also only a few hundred years old. Other countries where Kombucha is consumed, like Japan, China, Russia, and Germany, are far older than the USA.

I am apt to lean on age-old wisdom than I am to only take medical and scientific advice from a baby. I love my country and all the wonderful things it does, but if it weren't for profit, revenue, and regulation by corporations and pharmaceutical companies, I don't think it would have taken us 200 years to come up with a healthy "cure for cancer" that is inexpensive, easy to produce, and has no adverse side effects. I have witnessed first hand that this drink, when included in a larger regimen of healthy diet, helped me cure a virus in my own body that is responsible for causing cancer. This inspired me to write this book and share the wealth of Kombucha healing with you.

Kombucha, as it is widely known in English, has many names in other cultures. This word has its origins in Japanese and means "algae tea." However, when the brew was translated for English, it may have been confused with a type of drink in Japan that is made from the Kombu algae. "Kombucha" is not known by the Japanese to be the type of drink that English speakers call "Kombucha." The origins of the English translation are unknown as well as the origins of Kombucha itself.

Some say that the first documented use of Kombucha goes as far back as around 200 BC in the Qin dynasty of China. Some say that Kombucha is referenced in the Bible (Ruth 2:14) as a vinegar drink. Some say it was introduced to Japan by a Korean physician named Kombu, in about 400 AD. Some say it has been a popular household drink over the past century in parts of Russia where cancer is non-existent and longevity is high. Some say German physicians used the drink in the 19th century to cure a wide variety of ailments. I am certainly no expert on the history and creditability of historical sources for this delicious drink, but I *am* here to tell you how to enjoy and benefit from it in your own life.

I believe that, as long as your brew remains healthy, there are no adverse side effects to drinking Kombucha. You are more likely to experience benefits by welcoming this drink into your life, especially as a compassionate Kombucha brewer.

Here is an extensive list of ailments that Kombucha is said to have healed, cured, treated, or prevented. Again, these are only claims that have no concrete backup by the American scientific or medical industry. There is a gamut of scientific and medical research or personal claims on Kombucha from around the globe, but this is usually deemed inconclusive or discreditable by American standards. I leave it up to you to draw your own conclusions.

Ailments

AIDS {prolongs life of patients} : Anxiety : Arthritis : Asthma : Autoimmune Disorders : Cancer : Candida : Constipation : Depression : Diabetes : Eczema : Fibromyalgia : Flu and Colds : Gastrointestinal Disorders : High Blood Pressure : HPV and other STDs : Kidney Stones and Bladder Infections : Liver Toxicity : Migraines and Headaches : Obesity : Ulcers

So how can one simple drink that you can inexpensively create in your own home be thought of as a miracle cure-all? Here are some health benefits that are attributed to Kombucha.

Health Benefits

Promotes Healthy Cell Regeneration

Detoxification

Improves Energy

Improves Immune Function

Promotes Healthy Joints

Improves Metabolism

Promotes Healthy Intestinal Bacteria

It is said that Kombucha is antioxidant, probiotic, and contains many natural enzymes and acids that are healthy for the body. If Kombucha does, in fact, promote the above health benefits, than it is easy to see why any ailments having to do with a low immune system, mutated cells, joint pain, toxicity, unhealthy intestinal flora, low metabolism, and low energy can be alleviated by drinking it. If you improve many functions at once, it can drastically increase the quality of life for someone suffering from any of the above ailments.

This drink should be used in conjunction with other healthy lifestyle and diet choices, as well as treatment by medical professionals, in order to see the full benefits. It is not meant to be a miracle medicine, but you are welcome to try it out, experiment, and include it in your own regimen. You can experience good health, healing, and your own miracles by drinking Kombucha, regardless of the lack or abundance of "proof" that it promotes longevity, heals, and cures disease.

Tea Types & Health Benefits

Tea used for Kombucha is generally made from the *Camellia sinensus* plant. In order to make tea, the leaves may undergo several processes such as drying, steaming, and fermenting/oxidation. This list of tea is in order from least processed to most processed and is given along with their health benefits. By consulting this list, you can choose the type of tea that may be most appropriate for your healing desires.

White Tea

Immune boosting. Promotes healthy skin and anti-aging. Anti-cancer. Antimicrobial (alleviates viral, bacterial, and fungal infections).

Green Tea

Immune boosting. Cardiovascular support (alleviates heart disease, high blood pressure, and high cholesterol). Anti-cancer. Antimicrobial (alleviates viral, bacterial, and fungal infections).

Oolong Tea

Promotes healthy skin, teeth, and bones. Promotes mental acuity. Metabolism (for weight loss, diabetes, and obesity). Reduces stress and anxiety. Anti-cancer.

Black Tea

Cardiovascular support (alleviates heart disease, high blood pressure, and high cholesterol). Alleviates digestive and intestinal disorders. Anti-cancer. Alleviates asthma.

You can use other types of tea to make Kombucha but this is not highly recommended, especially for beginning brewers. It is good to have an extra healthy Scoby on hand if you choose to experiment with other types of tea, such as Rooibos and Herbal.

Herbs

The following is a list of herbs along with some of their health benefits. These can be added to your tea in their organic and dried form when you steep your tea before brewing. Herbs can add flavor and give your Kombucha an extra healing boost. I would recommend adding only 1-3 herbs, as too many herbs may result in a Kombucha that does not taste good. You may also need to experiment with flavors. Remember, your final Kombucha brew may taste different than the original steeped tea. It's always a good idea to have a healthy Scoby as a backup before you start experimenting with herbs.

Basil~ Antibacterial. Cardiovascular. Anti-cancer. Digestion. Relief for migraine and headache.

Cacao (use raw nibs)~ Antidepressant. Anti-cancer. Antioxidant. Cognitive function. Energy booster. Immune boosting.

Chamomile ~ Anti-stress and anti-anxiety. Anti-inflammatory. Menstrual health. Sleep, relaxation, and anti-insomnia.

Cinnamon ~ Anti-inflammatory. Antimicrobial. Cardiovascular support. Cognitive function.

Cloves ~ Anti-cancer. Antimicrobial. Anti-inflammatory. Immune boosting.

Fennel ~ Antimicrobial. Anti-anxiety. Digestion.

Echinacea ~ Antibacterial. Immune boosting.

Ginger ~ Antioxidant. Antimicrobial. Anti-inflammatory. Anti-cancer. Digestion. Immune boosting.

Goldenseal ~ Antimicrobial. Digestion. Immune boosting.

Lavender ~ Relief for migraine and headache. Antidepressant. Anti-stress and anti-anxiety. Antimicrobial.

Lemon Balm ~ Antidepressant. Digestion. Anti-stress and anti-anxiety. Sleep regulation and anti-insomnia.

Licorice Root ~ Antibacterial. Digestion. Anti-inflammatory.

Mugwort ~ Antibacterial. Digestion. Woman's reproductive health.

Peppermint (also spearmint and wintergreen) ~ Digestion. Anti-anxiety. Antibacterial. Anti-inflammatory. Cognitive function. Relief for migraine, headache, and sinus pressure. Men's reproductive health.

Vanilla ~ Anti-cancer. Antimicrobial. Antioxidant. Immune booster. Relaxation.

You can combine the health information in this chapter with the manifestation information in the next chapter to make a super healing brew of Kombucha.

By Allison Gee

Kombucha for Manifestation

Now that you are educated about Kombucha, we get to talk about the fun stuff! We're going to talk about using Kombucha as a companion in manifestation. Whether you want more money, true soulmate love, a better career, or to travel the world, I'm going to teach you how to turn your Kombucha into a real potion to help you attain your desires. Again, potions should be used in conjunction with helpful diet, lifestyle, mindset, emotional, and physical environments to receive the full benefits.

You may be wondering how a drink can help you do things like fall in love or attain more money, but when you understand the "science" behind it, this will make sense and you will be wondering why no one told you before. If you're going to be too analytical about it because everything you've ever known says you can't drink something to attain love and money, than you will be hindering your manifestation already. Just try it and see if it brings you results. You don't need to fully understand exactly how something works in order to receive the benefits from using it. You can take the tools you learn here and apply them to other parts of your life.

<u>Manifestation Basics</u>

There are some basic components to create a manifestation. It is important to understand these so you can apply them to your Kombucha brewing environment. The manner in which you brew your Kombucha, in addition to the basic brewing process, is what will create your potion.

Here are some of the different elements to create a manifestation:

Beliefs & Imagination

The beliefs that you have about your life and reality, whether conscious or subconscious, can make or break your ability to manifest. Imagination can overcome negative beliefs. For instance, if you don't believe a Kombucha potion will actually give you more money, just imagine that it does and you will accelerate your manifestation. Imagination can also bring in the creativity you need to create your own manifestation brewing formulas.

Thoughts & Intuition

You are in control of your thoughts. Sometimes it may feel like you are not, but if you have a thought you don't like, just think a bunch that you do. Practice exercising conscious control and modulation of your own thoughts. Having thoughts in alignment with your desired outcome will get you where you want to go. Sometimes intuition can be mistaken as a thought you made up in your head, so pay attention if thoughts come in that feel like they are too brilliant for you to make up only on your own. You may be receiving assistance from the ethers of the universe.

Feelings & Emotions

You also have control over your emotions. Again, if you have one you don't like, instill a bunch that you do like. Practice having conscious control and modulation of your own emotions. Utilize the other elements like imagination and sound if you are having challenges creating emotions for yourself. Having emotions in alignment with your desired outcome will help you bring in your manifestation. Feelings can be intuition too; you can have a feeling without having an emotion. Again, pay attention to feelings that seem too brilliant to only be your own.

Speech & Sound

Speech includes both the written word and spoken word. Speech is also a vibratory frequency of sound. You can use other sounds, like a pleasing piece of music, to bring your life into alignment with your desired outcome. Sound is powerful because its vibratory frequency can change the energetic makeup of a substance, like Kombucha.

Be conscientious of how you are speaking and practice the conscious control and modulation of your speech to be in alignment with your desired outcome. For instance, if you desire to be wealthy, do you go around telling people you are broke and poor? In this case, your desired outcome and your speech would be disharmonious, hindering your manifestation. Instead you might say that your money is healing or that you are working on manifesting more, even if that may not be a conventional way to speak to people in your life.

Actions & Will Power

Actions are how you exert yourself in the world in order to attain your desired outcome. It may also take some will power and alignment with the other basic elements to be able to do this effectively. For instance, if you desire more love in your life and you have been granted this book, do you just let it sit around on your shelf or digital device when you are finished reading without taking action, or do you start to take the steps one by one to brew yourself a Kombucha love potion? It may take some will power to go and do it, and it may take repeated action and experience to do it well. For some it may be easier than others.

At first it may feel like learning a new skill to consciously modulate and control your thoughts and emotions instead of just being reactionary. It's clear that we have not been raised, as a humanity, to be effective creators and manifestors. If we were, more of us would have the life we desire to live and get everything that we want in a harmonious, compassionate way that produces abundance for all life on Earth. Creating an elixir to drink for your love life is only fictional magic until you understand how it is done, you do it, and you experience the benefits. Are you ready? Here we go!

Manifestation Basics in Kombucha Brewing

Before you start creating Kombucha elixirs and potions, I recommend you attain a way to document your journey and results. Start a blog, buy a blank journal, open a document on your device; do something to record your benefits. It will give you something to read so you can track your progress. This is helpful during the challenging times when you feel like giving up, you start to think your efforts have been wasted, or you don't think it's working. Sometimes this happens in the manifesting process just before a breakthrough, and if you give in, the breakthrough doesn't happen. If you have something to hold yourself accountable that you need to document, a little light bulb will hopefully go off in your head when something happens that is in alignment with your desired outcome. If you don't have a method of documentation, you are more likely to ignore or discount an opportunity, situation, or occurrence as it arises.

Your current status quo of beliefs may attempt to rubber band you back into your habitual mode of operation when you strive to make a change and manifest something new. If you have any current feelings, beliefs, or thoughts that will hinder your manifestation, let go of them now. Don't listen to them! These voices sound like, "You can't do that. You can't have that. You don't deserve that. You're not good enough. This isn't working. Etc." Tell them you love them, thank them for speaking their opinion, and compassionately ask them to leave so you can get on with your manifestation. These are "lower vibratory" thoughts- thoughts that do not align with your desired outcome. They hinder or thwart your capabilities to manifest. Document if you notice you have a negative pattern somewhere. It will be a good clue as to what is stopping you so you can heal it. When you pass the challenges, you will create miracles.

Now that you know some basic elements of manifestation, you can use these elements to align your life with your desired vibratory frequency and create a Kombucha potion. Use the manifestation basics to create your ideal Kombucha brewing environment. This is great practice for consciously modulating these basic elements to create something- in this case, a Kombucha manifesting elixir. I have provided a suggestion of steps, but you are welcome to use your imagination to come up with your own.

Step 1: Using Thoughts & Imagination

Come up with a desired outcome that you have if you were to drink a magic potion and make it come true. If you need assistance in creating this desired outcome, use the area of life that you are least satisfied with right now. I encourage you to pick only one for your elixir. Choose from the following areas~

Love & Romance

Finances

Career

Health (This can be physical, mental, emotional, or spiritual health.)

Social Life

Family

Recreation & Entertainment

There are some guidelines to follow to create an empowered manifestation. Things are easier to manifest when you are specific and direct with your manifestation request. For instance, if you desire more money, come up with a specific amount. It is also more powerful to formulate the manifestation based on how you desire to experience life, rather than impose your desire on another person or thing. If it is an object that you desire, like a new car, state your desire for your "soulmate car" and get specific about the features, like the color and type. If you desire more romance in your life, come up with how you want to feel and experience that romance instead of saying who you want to have it with. The who is just a means to a desired vibratory frequency. The ethers of the universe often have something else in mind that is far better and beyond anything you thought you wanted in the first place. These guidelines make it easier to compassionately bring in your manifestation.

When you have a desired outcome, use some actions and written speech to document it on the first page of your journal. Again, pick an area of life, formulate a specific and direct phrase or statement that you want to come true after drinking your potion, and write it down. Congratulations! You have taken the first step on your manifesting journey.

You can use your thoughts and imagination from here on to create new elements for your Kombucha brewing environment that are in alignment with your desired outcome. Eventually you will use your thoughts and imagination to come up with your own unique brewing formulas that are special for you.

Step 2: Using Feelings & Emotions

While you are preparing your Kombucha to brew, imagine how you feel when you have your desired outcome, even if it feels like pretend at first. You may have to utilize the other elements to evoke these feelings. For example, if you desire a new car, use speech and say, "Woo hoo! I feel so happy that I have my new car," and start telling yourself all about it- the make, model, color, and where you drive it. This will certainly evoke some good feelings while you are boiling the water and steeping the tea.

Use positive feelings and emotions toward your Scoby every day. If it's love you want, just give that jar a hug and tell it how much you love it. This may sound silly, but a Scoby is a living organism, and like any living organism, it responds to the vibratory frequency in its immediate environment. Think of your heart center as a technology. Use your emotions to tell your Scoby what you want your life to bring by drinking the Kombucha it is making.

Step 3: Using Speech & Sound

Besides talking to your Scoby and your Kombucha, you can use words in other creative ways. Tape or write beautifully written words onto your brewing container. This gives you a nice visual reminder of your desired manifestation. It also helps the essence of the liquid align with your desired outcome.

You can play music to your brewing Kombucha. Find music that really evokes the feelings and experiences you desire to have after drinking your elixir. Be cautious though; if your music contains lyrics, you will want to make sure you listen to them all so you are clear on what kind of frequency you are telling your Kombucha to bring you. There are lots of lower vibratory lyrics and themes in music that you may not want to instill into yourself. I would recommend instrumental music, unless you have reviewed the whole song with a manifesting perspective before playing the music to your brewing Kombucha.

Step 4: Using Action & Will Power

You will use a lot of will power to perform the actions that create a positive environment for your brewing Kombucha. It may take will power to overcome lower vibratory thoughts and feelings along the way. I recommend doing something every day to create a positive environment for your brew that is in alignment with your desired outcome. You may need will power to do something every day for 7-14 days. With repeated practice, you will create a stronger elixir.

Every couple of weeks, you can take the actions of drinking your potion and documenting any effects you notice in your life. Document for 30 to 90 days after you start drinking your potion. You will re-brew it within that time and work on attaining your desired outcome. If you get a feeling from your internal compass of an inspired action to take that will bring you your manifestation, go for it. It is a fun and exciting adventure for you to see where life takes you after drinking your compassionate Kombucha elixir.

If challenging experiences arise during your manifesting journey, just take a deep breath and get curious. Ask yourself what you are learning from the experience, and ask yourself if this experience is aligning you with your desired outcome. Sometimes when we desire to make a positive change, old patterns, people, mindsets, emotions, and ways of being fall away to make room for this new manifestation. Experiences that may seem negative while they are happening can often be looked back upon as a positive experience after the occurrence is over.

Manifestation Elixir Recipes and Regimens

Here is a suggested list of elements to include in your brewing recipe or environment for each area of life listed in Step 1.

Recipe Key

Herbs: Can be placed in their dried form into your steeping tea or the plant can be placed beside your brew.

Luck Stones: These are good friends for brewing compassionate Kombucha. Place them beside your brew. You may have a bright idea to place them inside your brew, but I will leave it up to you to manage this. It can be less sanitary and more effort so I wouldn't recommend it until you are proficient at creating manifesting elixirs.

Elemental: This is a physical element of Earth, Water, Air, or Fire that you can incorporate in your brewing environment.

Room Area: This is the suggested area of the home or room to place your brew. The reference point is from standing at the entrance facing in. For instance, if the room area says "back left corner," you would stand at the entrance of your home or room, facing into the space, and place it in the back left corner. These room areas are derived from the corresponding areas of the Bagua Map according to Feng Shui. I may not know exactly how Feng Shui works, and it may not be a creditable science according to my country and culture, but I know that it is a science for many. Again, you don't always have to understand exactly how something works in order to enjoy the benefits of using it.

Sound: This is the suggested sound, tone, or note to play to your brew. I will leave it up to you to find pleasing music that evokes your desired outcome.

Love & Romance

Herbs: Rose. Jasmine. Lavender.

Luck Stones: Rose quartz. Ruby. Garnet.

Elemental: Fire- Safely burn a red candle. Water- Add a splash of rose water. Air- Burn some rose or jasmine incense. Earth- Put an orchid or lily beside your brew (do not eat it).

Room Area: Back right corner.

Sound: Pure love- Note F. Sexuality- Note C.

Finances

Herbs: Basil. Peppermint. Cloves. Cinnamon. Ginger.

Luck Stones: Jade. Aventurine. Amethyst. Fluorite. Emerald.

Elemental: Earth- Put a Jade or Mint plant beside your brew (do not eat Jade). Water- Put a fountain beside your brew. Air- Burn some sage and smudge around your brew. Fire- Safely burn a green candle.

Room Area: Back left corner.

Sound: Healing- Note C. Attaining- Note D.

Career

Herbs: Basil. Bergamot. Lavender.

Luck Stones: Citrine. Tiger Eye. Topaz.

Elemental: Earth- Place some acorns beside your brew. Water- Bless your brew by putting your index and middle finger into the liquid and make a wish. Air- Frankincense incense. Fire- Safely burn a green or orange candle.

Room Area: Entrance- work and job. Back side- reputation and legacy. Near left corner- knowledge, wisdom, and education.

Sound: Getting a job- Note D. Career success- Note E.

Health

Herbs: {Covered extensively in the Health and Healing chapter.}

Luck Stones: Amethyst. Clear Quartz. Sea salt crystals. Lapis Lazuli (spiritual and mental). Moonstone (women's health). Obsidian or Garnet (men's health). Hematite (cardiovascular).

Elemental: Earth- Put a large stone beside your brew. Water- Add a splash of lemon juice and honey. Air-

Diffuse some Rosemary oil. Fire- Safely burn a white candle.

Room Area: Left side- healing. Center- well-being, unity, and balance.

Sound: Physical- Note E. Emotional- Note F. Mental- Note A. Spiritual- Note B.

Social

Herbs: Apple. Lemon. Vanilla.

Luck Stones: Amber. Turquoise.

Elemental: Earth- Arbor Vitae wreath. Water- Add a splash of orange juice. Air- Honeysuckle incense. Fire- Safely burn a blue or yellow candle.

Room Area: Left side- community. Back side- reputation. Near right corner- helpful people.

Sound: Friendship- Note E. Communication- Note G.

Family

Herbs: Basil. Marjoram.

Luck Stones: Agate. Citrine.

Elemental: Earth- Put several pebbles in a ring around your brew. Water- Splash a little of your brew onto a water resistant family photo. Air- Myrrh incense. Fire-

If you have a functional fireplace in your home, light a cozy fire and bring your brew into the room.

Room Area: Left side- family life and community. Right side- children.

Sound: Fertility, loyalty, togetherness- Note C. Healing emotional matters- Note F.

Recreation & Entertainment

Herbs: Vanilla. Cacao. Coconut.

Luck Stones: Aventurine. Malachite.

Elemental: Earth- Place some sand near your brew. Water- Fill a small bowl with sea salt crystals, shells, and water. Air- Apple Blossom incense. Fire- Safely burn a blue or purple candle.

Room Area: Right side- creativity, fun, and entertainment. Near right corner- travel and adventure.

Sound: Fun- Note D. Travel- Note B.

The recipes in this chapter are a good suggested starting point for you to brew your own potions. You are free to use your creative imagination to come up with your own recipes and environmental elements. Use items in your recipe and brewing environment that are special to you. Don't forget to document the outcomes you observe in your life after drinking your potions.

Compassionate Kombucha

By Allison Gee

Let Food Be Thy Medicine

I would like to reiterate that it's important to use Kombucha potions along with a healthy lifestyle. When other elements of your life are healthy, it is easier to manifest your desires. As a holistic practitioner, I generally do my best to live a fairly healthy life. However, when I was diagnosed with a virus that I was told could possibly turn into cancer, I wanted to figure out how to heal it fast while my doctors prescribed that I "watch and wait." I wanted to figure out what to do that would be simple so I could implement it into my life, independent from medical attention, in case I contracted this ailment again. I remembered a famous saying,

"Let food be thy medicine." ~ Hippocrates

So I did, and I healed my abnormal cells within 3 months. I wanted to share with you, the diet that I used to heal my body. When you read this regimen, you may think it's so simple that it's common sense. However, for an average American like myself, it was challenging at first to implement because of the amount of unhealthy food that is ingrained in the average diet in my country. Now that I'm healed, I am no longer as strict with myself about continuing this diet, but I would recommend it if you have a prolonged mild or chronic ailment. If you want to adopt and incorporate more of these dietary elements into your life, I am sure it will bring you good health.

This "diet" is a regimen of food that helped me heal my body from a very common virus. This skin virus causes cancer and death for thousands of people, particularly women, each year. Although the chances of cancer are low, statistics on this virus say that 50%-80% of people will contract this virus sometime in their lifetime {provided they have ever had sex}. My doctor told me it was 100% of people. Many of them will never know they have it, are carrying it, or are spreading it around because it often produces no visible symptoms or pain, and some will never know they have it until it turns into cancer.

Healthy sexuality is important for being an effective, compassionate creator and manifestor. However, sexuality in my country and culture is a sensitive subject because so many of us have had lower vibratory experiences, beliefs, thoughts, emotions, speech, and actions programmed into us about this important facet of life. Risk of contracting a virus that could turn into cancer is just one example. It may even be bold of me to publish my relationship with this virus, for the first time, in my book about Kombucha. However, this relationship and my healing inspired me to write this book and help others use something simple to cure what ails them.

Just like a computer with a virus, I believe we can wipe it away and deprogram our world of both cancer and unhealthy sexuality. If you can grasp the scope of what I am proposing, than you will know that curing HPV and cervical cancer is just a small feat. I refuse to believe that "there is no cure," but if we found out what the cure is, it may take someone other than a western medical doctor to point out that the cure is at the grocery store. I'm also fairly sure that none of my doctors would think it was anything revolutionary if I told them I cured myself with food. No one at my checkup thought it was anything miraculous when I went in with abnormal cells and went back with no abnormal cells a few months later. I know it is easy to discount because this thing comes and goes and sometimes your immune system clears it out on its own, but I am fairly certain my change in diet helped it go away.

I know that many people are not educated about this virus and many people will not be aware of it until they are told they have it. Being safe and responsible with your sexuality doesn't necessarily protect you from this virus because it is spread through skin to skin contact. It is highly likely that you will contract this virus sometime in your lifetime. One of the best lessons I've leaned over my two and a half year journey with this virus is that it's good to be educated, but there is no need to get emotional or paranoid. I wanted to gift you this knowledge and wisdom so you don't freak out (like I did at first) if you are diagnosed with a disease. Let food be thy medicine!

Goddess Allison's Healing Diet

This 3 month diet and regimen is what worked for me based on my own internal compass. It was a bit challenging for the first month, but after that it was easy and my body no longer craved unhealthy food. There were times I let myself slip up on my diet, especially for special occasions, but the regular habit of being food conscientious was a beneficial learning and healing experience. If you chose to use a regimen of food to help your body cure cancer, viruses, and other disease, I encourage you to use your own discretion about what is best for your body. Modulate this diet to fit your own desired outcome, and use this information along with treatment and care by medical professionals. A Kombucha healing potion here and there can help you too!

Basic Regimen

~Make sure your food is all organic and minimally processed!

You may find that your food bill would increase to purchase organic food or to purchase many of the items in this diet all at once. As I like to tell people, "Expensive is a matter of perspective." Instead focus on the value you are receiving from the food- it's healthy and it will help your body heal. It also took a lot of time and energy to grow, package, and transport so that you can eat it in the comfort of your own home. Now that's value! If you can't acquire everything all at once, just do your best and purchase what you feel your body needs most.

~Make sure you are drinking plenty of fluids.

Try for half your body weight in ounces per day, but if that's too much, just do your best. {For instance, if you weigh 100 lbs, drink 50 oz of water per day}.

~Primarily Vegetables

My healing diet consisted primarily of vegetables. I ate lots of kale, spinach, carrots, lentils, sweet potatoes, etc. I often ate a green smoothie for breakfast with vegetables and fruit, especially on the weekdays.

Legumes are vegetables but may be considered seeds too. I would recommend eating beans in their most natural and minimally processed form. Soak them, boil them up, add some salt, and mix them in with other healing foods in this diet.

~Some Fruit

I ate some fruit, especially fruit high in Vitamin C and antioxidants. Pineapple, blueberries, acaí berries, strawberries, goji berries, citrus fruit like oranges and lemons, etc.

~Some Nuts and Seeds

Soaked/sprouted and minimally processed is best because it is easiest for your body to digest. Many seeds and nuts have enzymes so they can be passed through the digestive system to be carried away, excreted, and planted far from their origin. Soaking the seeds and nuts in water for 12-24 hours breaks down these enzymes and wakes up their natural process for growing. When you are healing you want your body to use energy with maximum efficiency, and eating nuts and seeds that come to you with oils, salt, sugar, and other additives is not the most ideal choice.

I ate chia seeds, pumpkin seeds, cashews, sesame seeds, sunflower seeds, almonds, and quinoa. I did not eat any peanuts because I don't care for them much and my work environment was peanut free, so that dietary element was my personal choice. Some nuts and seeds can also be considered grains (like flaxseed) or be confused with being a grain (like quinoa).

~Some Grains

Make sure your grains and seeds are minimally processed. Just because you are eating a food that contains "whole grains" or "whole grain wheat" does not necessarily mean that your body will have a fun and easy time digesting those things for nutrients. Whole grain wheat flour has undergone some kind of process to turn it into this substance, and unless you ground the wheat yourself, you are removed from knowing the conditions of this process. Processed corn and wheat are main ingredients in a large amount of food. This can be one reason why minimally processed and no processed food can be challenging to implement and navigate in your healing diet.

The main grain I ate was brown or black rice. White rice is more processed and less nutritious than brown or black, but I did eat white rice a few times when it was the only option (like when you go out to eat). Other grains I ate were farro, oats/oatmeal, and millet.

~Minimal Gluten

I had heard it is more work for your body to process gluten, so I didn't eat bread, not even gluten free bread because that can be a processed food. I tried to stay away from things that had been made with flour and wheat, and I tried not to eat any other processed "gluten free" foods. I wanted to eat food that was easy for my body to digest while being highly nutritious and in its most natural form. When you cook or bake things together, this can alchemically change the content of the food and possibly make it more difficult for your body to process. Unless you do the cooking and baking yourself, you are more removed from the quality of ingredients in your food and the process it underwent before you eat it.

~Minimal Meat

I only ate small animal meat because I had heard from a nutritionist that small animal proteins are easier for the body to process, and even then I only ate meat once or twice per month. I ate grass fed lamb and wild caught salmon I purchased at my local farmer's market. I love making sushi and didn't want to give it up for my healing diet, but I replaced some of the ingredients with healthier alternatives- turned sushi rice into black rice, tuna into salmon, and raw grass fed beef into raw grass fed lamb. Several years ago a friend of mine, who favors a primal diet, proposed that I eat more raw meat, as long as it was grass fed and most likely sourced from my local farmers. The idea intrigued me, and after my own research to deduce this would be safe, I had been using raw grass fed beef as an option in my sushi ever since.

I did eat eggs rarely on my healing diet, but I did not eat chicken meat. I did not feel I wanted to eat chicken or other poultry on my diet, but you can choose what your body says to you. I did not eat any pig meat on my diet and I only ate cow meat once.

I remember only one time during my healing diet when I slipped up for a special occasion and ate a cheese burger with a bun, cheddar cheese, a hamburger patty (cow), a slice of tomato, and some lettuce, with no sauces. By this time I had been on my healing diet for over a month. I did my best to make sure the ingredients were in their best form, like cheddar cheese instead of American Cheese {which isn't actually cheese anyway} and no sauces like ketchup because they often contain high fructose corn syrup. I talked to my body before hand to tell it that this was coming and I promised myself that I was going to feel joyful about this choice {instead of guilty}. My stomach still felt a bit queasy about an hour later, but I just laid down for a rest and felt better. It was a strange lesson to learn that, just like "American Cheese," the average American diet and typical American food that I had grown so accustomed to eating, no longer felt like healing or healthy food substances.

~Minimal Dairy

I only ate yogurt and kefir a few times over the 3 months because I had read that cultured and fermented foods were good for immune boosting. I did not drink any milk or eat much cheese, but I would say that raw milk and some artisan cheese would be safer to readily incorporate in your healing diet than processed milk and cheese. Make sure your yogurt and kefir are <u>unsweetened</u>, all natural, minimally processed, and don't come with additives.

You can add raw honey or fresh organic fruit on your own.

I replaced butter with raw coconut oil in my cooking.

~No refined sugar and no sweetener additives!

The only refined sugar I allowed was white sugar that I was using to make Kombucha, just because I still had a huge bag laying around. I would recommend using organic cane juice crystals though. This was also one of the most challenging things to navigate during my diet because so much of the food in my culture has been unnecessarily sweetened.

~No processed food!!!

Basically if it had more than a few ingredients, I didn't eat it. I especially didn't eat anything that had ingredients I didn't know how to pronounce. I never thought I'd turn into one of those people who checks the ingredient label on everything, but there I was in the store, suddenly very aware of anything that I was putting into my body because my desired outcome was to cure a cancer causing virus!

Eat Plenty of Immune Boosting Foods:

~Kombucha

I heard it was healthy when I was reading about immune boosting foods. Since I like making and drinking it anyway, I figured this would be easy to incorporate. I increased my intake to at least 1 cup per day. It wasn't until the last month of my diet that I started to get creative and compassionately think of my Kombucha drink as a magic potion. I wanted to share my diet and success, but as this diet includes the frequent ingestion of Kombucha, I wrote this book as a companion to those who may chose to implement this diet into their lifestyle. If you like to drink Kombucha regularly, it's much more fun and economical to make your own.

~1 Clove of Garlic per day

I ate one raw clove on an empty stomach, about 30 min before breakfast because I heard it was more potent for immune boosting when eaten alone.

~Shiitake Mushrooms

I love growing shiitakes anyway and I learned they have many immune boosting and healing properties. I ate some on the weekends once every two weeks when my mushroom growing kit had blossomed. Reishi mushrooms are also good for immune boosting. You can purchase a shiitake mushroom growing kit on the internet.

~Ginger

Ginger is great for immune boosting. I bought some ginger beer from my local farmer's market and drank it about once per month (it is a non-alcoholic drink). I also put raw ginger into stir fry. Some people like it in their green smoothies.

~Turmeric, Cumin, & Cinnamon

Like garlic and ginger, these foods are naturally made to keep the plant alive, repel pests, and ward off microbial infections. Use the advantages of nature! I had read that turmeric and cumin are good for healthy cell regeneration, and some claim that turmeric and cumin can cure cancer. I often sprinkled turmeric on my rice, meat, or vegetables and sprinkled cinnamon into my oatmeal.

~Green Tea

I ate the tea leaves by swallowing 5-7 Jasmine Green Tea Pearls per day. I had heard that drinking a cup of green tea was healthy for the immune system, but I decided it would be more potent for my body if I ate the leaves instead.

~Raw Cacao

This is a food that contains flavonoids, which are helpful to the body for health and healing. Cacao nibs are great. Make sure your cacao is not sweetened. If you can't get raw cacao, buying 100% cacao unsweetened baker's chocolate and adding dates, raisins, or a bit of raw honey is a good alternative. I found that eating chocolate in it's most natural form can trick your brain into thinking you are eating junk food, and it helped suppress challenging cravings that I first experienced after implementing this diet.

I celebrated my birthday during my diet, and I wanted to figure out a good healthy alternative to cake so I mixed 100% cacao unsweetened baker's chocolate with dates and eggs to bake the most healthy "brownies" I've ever eaten. That was it, brownies with only 3 ingredients!

~Raw Honey

If you want a little sweet, this is a nice addition, but don't go crazy just because your body is craving sugar. Honey also has antimicrobial properties. It is thought that adding honey and lemon with your tea is healing. Raw honey from a source like your local farmer's market is generally a better alternative to sweetener for the healing diet than commercially processed honey.

~High Quality Oils

I read that high quality, organic, minimally processed oils are good for the immune system. This means you can incorporate extra virgin olive oil and raw coconut oil into your healing diet. I used these in my cooking and food preparation instead of butter. I also hear it is healthy to eat a spoonful straight.

I had heard cod liver oil was good for skin health, and I was dealing with a skin virus. I took one capsule once per week or once every few days for the first couple months. I didn't make it a point to take it every day like I did with folic acid, garlic, Kombucha, and Green Tea leaves. This was one of the only "dietary supplements" I used.

Other Herbs and Supplements I used:

I incorporated the following based on the specific ailment that I was healing, but I encourage you to find healthy alternatives specific to your own healing needs.

~ 800 mcg of Folic Acid per day

I had read this supplement was good for women, like myself, who are on birth control and desire to promote healthy cell regeneration. Besides cod liver oil, this was the only "dietary supplement" I used during my healing diet.

~ Herbal Suppositories

These were 5 herbal vaginal suppositories, generally done once per week, as I was healing a skin virus on my cervix.

Lifestyle:

~I don't generally drink, and I have never smoked. I did not drink alcohol during this diet. I would say an occasional glass of wine would be more healthy than most other alcoholic drinks if you like your drinks. If you habitually smoke and drink alcohol, I would recommend you do your very best to decrease your intake as much as you can while you are on this diet.

~I was making a big transition in my life, but I would recommend minimal stress.

~Exercise is also good, even if it's just a good walk every day. I walked to and from work every weekday for a total of about 20 minutes per day.

~I did not have sex while I was on my diet. I wanted to see if this regimen worked without that factor of risk. When I started my diet, it had been at least 90 days since I had done such a thing anyway, so I figured I was a good test subject to try this out (some sexually transmitted ailments can take a while before they produce symptoms). This was specific for my unique situation, but I recommend that a healthy sexual lifestyle is important for healing and manifestation.

For the third time in my life, I received an abnormal pap smear in mid December of 2014- LSIL, positive for high risk HPV. I had already undergone one Leep procedure {to cut it out of my body}. I decided to make it my New Year's resolution to drastically alter my diet for 3 months, following the regimen in this chapter, to see if the virus went away. I was on this diet from mid January to mid April 2015.

By mid April of 2015, when I went for my colposcopy, the virus was gone! A colposcopy is a follow up check in that is recommended to women after receiving an abnormal pap smear. The cells on my cervix were normal so I didn't need a biopsy, as I had twice in the past. My colposcopy was more delayed than my doctor recommended, but I knew there would be minimal risk to me by waiting 3 months and, due to scheduling, mid April was the soonest appointment I could attend when I called the doctor in March.

I did not tell my doctor that I had changed my diet and that may be the reason no abnormal cells were found on my cervix only a few months after my abnormal pap smear. To a doctor, this result is no miracle and disclosing such a thing would probably not be amazing. For the medical world, this would be easily discountable because this virus commonly "comes and goes," there is "no cure" for this virus, and diet is not related to HPV, but for me this was my cure. I had been dealing with this virus for over two years, and I was looking for something to do to just make it go away. If I ever run across it again, I will not hesitate to implement this diet and regimen!

Healing Diet Conclusion

I do not believe there would be adverse side effects in implementing this diet for your own life. If anything, you are more likely to experience good health and healing by adopting elements of this diet. If someone you know has cancer, a virus, chronic bacterial or fungal infection, or any ailment related to joint pain, toxicity, unhealthy intestinal flora, low metabolism, and low energy, please share this information with them!

About the Author

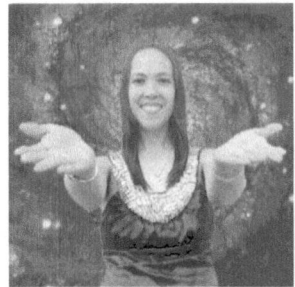 *Goddess Allison* is a manifestation mentor. She helps people become their own genie and make their wishes come true. To download a free PDF of the last chapter of this book, please visit the website below.

If you have enjoyed this book and would like to give feedback, provide a testimonial, contact the author, or book Allison for an event (workshop, retreat, media, speaking engagement, convention, etc.), please visit:

www.goddessallison.com

www.ingramcontent.com/pod-product-compliance
Lightning Source LLC
Chambersburg PA
CBHW020400290526
45785CB00005B/2375